Social and Emotional Well-Being

**Also in the Growing, Growing Strong:
A Whole Health Curriculum for Young Children Series**

Body Care

Fitness and Nutrition

Safety

Community and Environment

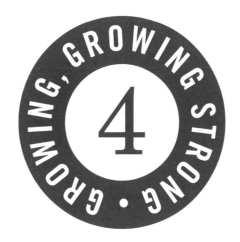

A Whole Health Curriculum for Young Children

Social and Emotional Well-Being

Third Edition

Connie Jo Smith
Charlotte M. Hendricks
Becky S. Bennett

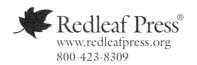

Redleaf Press®
www.redleafpress.org
800-423-8309

Published by Redleaf Press
10 Yorkton Court
St. Paul, MN 55117
www.redleafpress.org

First edition published 1997. Second edition 2006. Third edition 2014.
Cover design by Jim Handrigan
Cover photograph by Blend Images Photography/Veer
Interior design by Percolator
Typeset in Stone Informal, Matrix Script, and Trade Gothic
Illustrations by Chris Wold Dyrud
Photograph on page 49 by Blend Images Photography/Veer
Printed in the United States of America
20 19 18 17 16 15 14 13   1 2 3 4 5 6 7 8

Library of Congress Cataloging-in-Publication Data
Smith, Connie Jo.
  Growing, growing strong : a whole health curriculum for young children. Social and emotional well-being /
Connie Jo Smith, Charlotte M. Hendricks, and Becky S. Bennett. — Third edition.
    pages cm
  Summary: "Children's social and emotional skills form a critical foundation for learning and wellness that
guide them into adulthood and influence how they deal with both successes and adversity in life. These activities
support children as they learn about self-esteem, emotions and feelings, family and friends, and changes in life"
— Provided by publisher.
  ISBN 978-1-60554-243-0 (pbk.)
  ISBN 978-1-60554-334-5 (e-book)
  1. Health education (Preschool)—United States. 2. Health education (Elementary)—United States. 3. Life
skills—Study and teaching (Preschool)—United States. 4. Life skills—Study and teaching (Elementary)—United
States. 5. Self-esteem in children—Study and teaching (Preschool)—United States. 6. Self-esteem in children—
Study and teaching (Elementary)—United States. 7. Emotions—Study and teaching (Preschool)—United States.
8. Emotions—Study and teaching (Elementary)—United States. 9. Curriculum planning—United States.   I. Hendricks, Charlotte Mitchell, 1957- II. Bennett, Becky S., 1954- III. Title. IV. Title: Social and emotional well-being.
  LB1140.5.H4S647 2014
  372.37—dc23
                                                                    2013023390

Printed on acid-free paper

Contents

Acknowledgments

We would like to express heartfelt appreciation to our talented, hardworking, and ever-positive editor, Kyra Ostendorf. This book is much richer for her ideas, guidance, and smiles—those given in person and those that arrived through electronic communication ;-). Thanks to Elena Fultz and Grace Fowler, interns at Redleaf Press, who assisted in technical editing. We are grateful to David Heath for his initial editing support and encouragement. And, of course, we want to acknowledge all the individuals we have had professional encounters with over the years, as each contact has helped us grow and has enhanced our work.

Introduction

Young children are better able to cope with their ever-changing world, to overcome obstacles, and even to thrive and grow into emotionally healthy adults if they are provided opportunities to build their self-awareness and confidence. Caregivers can play an important role in helping children celebrate their individual differences, as well as develop acceptance and understanding of how each individual possesses differences, strengths, and abilities. Assisting children in recognizing and building on their individual strengths and recognizing those of others will allow each child to develop both appreciation of others and a sense of self-worth and confidence, key traits for social and emotional development addressed within this curriculum.

As children engage with the world around them, they will experience many emotions, some of which they will have more or less difficulty in handling. Through this curriculum, you can help each child identify and express feelings at a level suitable to her language skills and development, adding to her self-awareness and confidence. Each new experience and the resulting feelings can be confusing for a child. As children learn about themselves and explore their surroundings, you can support them by providing factual information and by helping them cope with and express their feelings in an appropriate manner.

This curriculum will also help children identify their family members and friends and begin to understand their own roles in these relationships. Young children generally think of their family as the people who live under the same roof with them. Their primary caregiver may be a father, mother, grandparent, sibling, aunt, uncle, stepparent, foster parent, or other guardian. In addition, many children have extended families and may have homes in more than one place. A child's sense of belonging in a family and home may be defined in a variety of ways. Regardless of the makeup, size, number, or location of those each child considers "family," this curriculum will encourage exploration and acceptance of a wide variety of living situations and families.

Curriculum topics include self-esteem, emotions and feelings, family, friends, and change in children's lives. Activities and resources will help children learn to appreciate themselves and others, begin to recognize various family structures and cultures, explore friend and family relationships, and develop coping mechanisms for dealing with change and difficult events in their lives.

Each chapter covers one topic and starts with an overview that includes suggested interest area materials, learning objectives, vocabulary words to introduce and use (which should include vocabulary words in the languages spoken by the families of children in the class), supports for creating the learning environment, and suggestions for evaluating children's understanding of the topic. The overview is followed by activity ideas. Icons appear with each activity to identify the areas of development and learning integrated into the activity:

= Arts

= Science

= Language

= Social Emotional

= Math

= Technology

= Physical

Each chapter concludes with a family information page and a take-home family activity page, both of which can be photocopied from the book and distributed to families. These pages can also be downloaded from the Growing, Growing Strong page at www.redleafpress.org for electronic sharing or printing.

INTEREST AREA MATERIALS

Dramatic Play

two or more no-longer-working telephones

unbreakable hand mirrors

full-length unbreakable mirrors

dolls that cry or laugh

close-up photographs of faces showing a variety of ethnicities and ages

plastic, silk, or dried flower centerpieces

suitcases

luggage carts

empty boxes for packing

family photos

Blocks

toy people, including adults and children

plastic or silk flowers for hauling and props

a variety of unbreakable mirrors

toy moving trucks

tiny boxes for moving

Table Toys

board games requiring two or more players

puzzles showing faces

lacing cards

Transformers

Lego blocks

toy people

dollhouse people

dollhouse furniture

Art

textured objects for rubbings

charcoal

colored chalk

plastic or silk flowers to incorporate into art

yarn

beads

magazine pages of people's faces for collages

Language Arts

puppets

copies of birth and death certificates

headstone pictures or catalogs

funeral programs or bulletins from a memorial service

posters of the life cycle of butterflies

clothing catalogs

recreational magazines and brochures

friendship greeting cards (cut off the signature page from used cards)

Library

You're All My Favorites by Sam McBratney

Pete the Cat: I Love My White Shoes by Eric Litwin

Knuffle Bunny: A Cautionary Tale by Mo Willems

The Family Book by Todd Parr

"I Have a Little Problem," Said the Bear by Heinz Janisch

Changes by Anthony Browne

Science/Math

butterfly garden kit

ladybug-, frog-, praying mantis-, sea monkey-, or earthworm-growing kits

pictures of optical illusions

tape measures

training wheels

magic trick supplies

Outdoors

rocking boats

double slides

riding toys for two

wagons

balls

beanbags

pillowcases or sacks for three-legged races

Technology

weather radio

listening games

laughing boxes

Sand, Water, and Construction

soil for burying things

hand trowel or shovel

plastic, silk, or dried flowers for arranging

stones

food coloring and eyedroppers

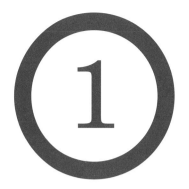

There's Something Special about Me!

LEARNING OBJECTIVES

- Children will identify characteristics they like about themselves.
- Children will identify skills they have and things they want to learn.
- Children will demonstrate self-help skills, including identifying clothing preferences.

How responsive and accepting adults are with children helps determine if the children learn to like or dislike themselves. A key element in working with children is learning to respect their level of capability and effort. Regardless of how long it takes or how recognizable the product is, a child may put a great deal of effort and pride into an activity, such as completing a puzzle or painting a picture. Help children feel good about themselves and their abilities by recognizing their efforts. Offer smiles, hugs, or words such as "I really like the colors you used!" or "You really worked hard on that!" Encourage individuality in children's work. The sky may not be blue and the grass may be bright pink, but the painting reflects the child's work and creativity. It is okay if a child draws a snowman surrounded by grass or paints flowers on a snow scene.

As a teacher, try to find a balance between accepting current abilities and challenging children to learn and develop new skills. Children will most naturally develop feelings of self-worth and confidence if you take time to interact with them, answer questions, provide information, give positive feedback, and supply a variety of opportunities for new experiences and practice.

5

Every child should feel appreciated every day. Greet children upon arrival, get on children's eye level to talk with them, and say children's names when you respond to them.

Maintain an attitude of guidance and feedback when a child exhibits inappropriate behavior. Let children know that it is the action or behavior that is unacceptable, not them. Additionally, assist the child in finding a more appropriate means of expression. Responding in this way allows children to continue feeling accepted and secure enough to try new things and develop new skills.

VOCABULARY

abilities	cheerful	kind	skills
accept	creative	leader	style
alike	different	like	talents
appreciate	favorite	performance	weight
athletic	height	proficient	
awaits turns	helpful	respect	
capable	interests	shares	

CREATING THE ENVIRONMENT

- Hang unbreakable mirrors and photographs of children at their eye level.
- Display children's artwork and projects.
- Label children's cubbies with their names and/or photographs.
- Include both quiet and busy interest areas and a variety of activities that allow children with a range of abilities and interests to succeed. Allow children to choose the interest area they wish to visit, and be sure to include materials that reflect each child's race, ethnicity, and cultural background. As time passes, add materials based on the interests children show and materials that will provide different challenges and allow success as children develop.

EVALUATION

- Do children seem to like themselves?
- Do children talk about what they can do?
- Do children try new things?
- Do children talk about clothing preferences (for example, a favorite shirt or color preference)?
- During pretend play, do children demonstrate self-help skills when dressing dolls (for example, with a zipper or buttons)?

CHILDREN'S ACTIVITIES

I Can Do This

Have children think of some activity they each really like to do or think they do well. Examples may include kicking a ball, working a puzzle, singing a song, telling a story, buttoning their clothes, drawing a picture, counting, or helping another. Ask the children to draw, demonstrate, or talk about the activity. They can display their picture for the group to see, show the group something they do well, teach other children how to do something, or talk to the group about something they can do. Encourage the group to show appreciation and acceptance of each thing a child contributes. Help the children understand that more than one person can be really good at an activity.

MATERIALS

- markers, crayons, chart paper, drawing paper, and props children need for their demonstrations

OTHER IDEAS

- Make a self-help checklist for each child, and include skills like brushing teeth, combing hair, washing hands, putting on shoes, putting on a coat, zipping clothes, and tying shoes. Read the chart to each child individually, and ask which of the tasks the child knows how to do already. Help the child check off those tasks.

- Invite family members to visit and tell about something they do well or something their child does well.

- Read and discuss *Harold and the Purple Crayon*, 50th Anniversary Edition, by Crockett Johnson. Talk about all of the things Harold can do with his purple crayon.

- Play, sing, and talk about "Shining Like a Star" by Laura Doherty.

  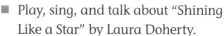

Talent Show

Have each child choose one special skill or talent to present in a show for families, another classroom, or a community group. Help children identify a wide range of talents and skills they may have, including drawing, running, using a computer, playing rhythm band instruments, building with blocks, making up songs or stories, and using a hammer. Some children may prefer to perform alone, and others may want to perform with friends or family members. Allow children to arrange a stage space, make invitations and tickets, practice their talents, make props, or design costumes for the show. Invite local media to attend, take photos to submit to media, or place photographs from the event on the program's website. Remember to obtain parent permission prior to their child's image or name being included for media purposes, including social media such as Facebook.

MATERIALS

- props and costumes, music, space for staging the show, paper, markers, paint, and signs

OTHER IDEAS

- Invite school employees, community leaders, and family members to visit the classroom and show their talents. Teach the children how to be a polite and appreciative audience during the performances and to clap afterwards. Follow up by helping children identify skills and talents they have similar to or different from those of the performing guests.

- Play, sing, and talk about "Dancing Pants" by In the Nick of Time and "Do My Thing" by Grenadilla.

- Read and discuss these or other books about talent shows: *Talent Show Scaredy-Pants* by Abby Klein, *Jack's Talent* by Maryann Cocca-Leffler, *The Talent Show* by Jo Hodgkinson, and *Albertine's Got Talent!* by Shena Power.

- Read and discuss *I Can Do It! A First Look at Not Giving Up* by Pat Thomas, or other books about learning new things and persistence.

"About Me" Display

Designate a space in the classroom for each child to set up a display, which may be in a box, on a tabletop, or posted on a bulletin board. The display might include a favorite toy or a picture of it, photos of her family, a list of things she can do, a drawing of something she likes about herself, or other items of importance to her. Allow the children to add to their displays for several days. At the end of that time, record the children talking about or explaining items in their "About Me" display or box. Let them invite family and friends to see or hear the recording. With parent permission, recordings could be included on classroom or program websites.

MATERIALS

- markers, paper, tape, poster board, favorite items, and a designated space for each child's display

OTHER IDEAS

- Read and discuss *What I Like about Me* by Allia Zobel Nolan.

- Play, sing, and talk about the songs "Be Yourself" by Grenadilla, "The Same as Me" by Grenadilla, "I Love My Toes" by the Cat's Pajamas, "That Would Be You" by the Cat's Pajamas, and "Free to Be . . . You and Me" by Marlo Thomas and Friends.

- Create a class chart with each child's name down the left side and traits (such as cheerful, helpful, kind, listens, creative, waits turns, shares, athletic, and musical) across the top. Help children understand each characteristic listed, and let them identify the ones they believe reflect who they are. Show them where to mark on the chart the characteristics that are theirs. Ask children which of the traits selected they like best.

- Create a class chart with each child's name down the left side and physical characteristics (such as eye color, hair color, hair length, skin color, shoe size, height, and so on) across the top. Help children understand each characteristic listed, and let them identify the ones that reflect who they are. Show them where on the chart to mark the characteristics that are theirs. Ask children which characteristic they like best of those selected.

I'm a Leader

Allow children to take turns being the leader during various transition times and activities. As leader, they might start a song with your prompting, be the leader of the line, or serve as the helper of the day. Select children to lead based on their interests and abilities so that all can shine in their leadership role, whether they are being the band director as other children play rhythm band instruments, greeting guests who enter the room, or distributing napkins for everyone. Ask children what they think they did best as a leader.

MATERIALS

- prop to make the leader look or feel special (baton, crown, cape)

OTHER IDEAS

- Read and discuss *Tillie and the Wall* by Leo Lionni or other books about leadership.

- Play the traditional game Follow the Leader, and give each child the opportunity to both follow and lead. Discuss the role of leadership and how important it is for the leaders to consider the followers.

- Invite leaders from the school or community to talk about their jobs as leaders and how being a leader makes them feel.

- Read and discuss *A Day's Work* by Eve Bunting.

My Favorites

Designate a "My Favorites" day for each child. On the designated day, allow the child to bring a favorite toy, wear a favorite article of clothing, have a favorite story read, lead a favorite game, sing a favorite song, and sit in a favorite spot. Encourage discussion about why the child likes these things, and show appreciation and support for the choices.

MATERIALS

 materials identified by children

OTHER IDEAS

 Have a series of "My Favorite" days, each with a different focus, such as "Favorite Book Day" or "Favorite Thing about Myself Day." Encourage each child to select his favorite for the day and share it with the group.

 Create a chart of favorite games you play with the children. Put their names down the side and the game names across the top. Each child then places an *X* in the correct box to indicate a favorite game. With the children, count the votes for each game, and let them know which game is the favorite of the most people in the group.

 Read and discuss *You're All My Favorites* by Sam McBratney. Talk about how sometimes there is not a single favorite and how people can like several things (or people) in equal amounts.

 Play, sing, move to the music, and talk about the song "My Favorite Things" by Julie Andrews or some other performer. Encourage children to think about their own favorite things about themselves and share them.

Developing Designs

Show children a few pieces of clothing, each of a very different style, and encourage them to talk about the similarities and differences. Ask children what kinds of clothes they like and why. Explain that someone designed their clothes and that some people do this as their job. Tell them that one way to design clothes is to draw an idea first and then cut it out of cloth. Show them sewing patterns. See if they want to design a piece of clothing for a doll or themselves. Help children think about the steps in creating clothes, and provide them with materials to produce their new designs.

  ♥

MATERIALS

- a variety of clothing items, sewing patterns, measuring tape, pencils, tissue paper, scissors, fabric, and accessories

OTHER IDEAS

- Visit a sewing factory or a sewing class to see the equipment and samples of clothes made.

    💻

- Invite a tailor who makes clothes or performs alterations to come speak to the class about his job. Encourage the visitor to show some of the tools he uses to do his job, and see if he will measure a few children to show them what a fitting is. Alternatively, watch a video clip of a tailor and discuss it.

   💬 ➕

- Read and role-play *Jesse Bear, What Will You Wear?* by Nancy White Carlstrom, *Pete the Cat: I Love My White Shoes* by Eric Litwin, or another book about children's clothes.

   💬 ♥

- Encourage children to create a group collage using pictures of clothes from catalogs and magazines. Initiate discussions about the purpose, styles, and sizes of clothing.

   💬 ♥

FAMILY INFORMATION

THERE'S SOMETHING SPECIAL ABOUT ME!

Children who feel good about themselves are better able to cope with daily situations. Children develop self-esteem by receiving praise and encouragement from family members and through love and security provided at home.

No child excels at everything. Some children can run fast or jump high, others easily learn to read or write, and some can tie their own shoes at an early age. But some tasks are more difficult for individual children.

Assure your child that it is okay if he or she cannot do something. Usually practice will develop or improve skills. Acknowledge your child's skills as they develop, and notice her or his efforts to learn new skills. Recognize your child's accomplishments, such as putting away a toy, getting dressed, throwing a ball, or reading or looking through a book with you.

EVERY CHILD IS SPECIAL

Help children feel good about themselves and their abilities by recognizing them. Offer smiles, hugs, and words, such as "I like the colors you used!" or "You really worked hard on that!"

Encourage individualization. Children may color the sky green and the grass pink, and that is okay. Some children love to sing and make up their own songs. Other children dance to their own music and their own beat.

You can help your child feel good about himself or herself. In front of a mirror, have your child repeat affirmations, such as "My favorite thing about me is (my hair, my smile, how smart I am)" and "I sure can (whistle, draw, skip) well."

FAMILY ACTIVITY

Help your child finish the sentences below by circling choices in the column on the right.
Discuss other things your child likes about herself or himself and that he or she can do.

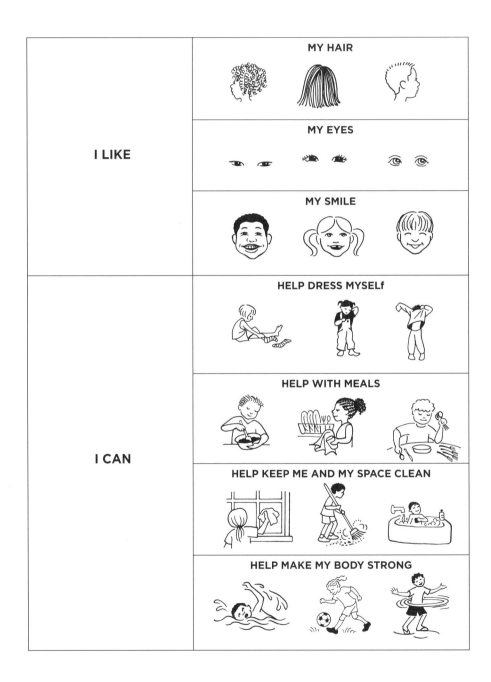

From *Social and Emotional Well-Being* by Connie Jo Smith, Charlotte M. Hendricks, and Becky S. Bennett,
© 2014. Published by Redleaf Press, www.redleafpress.org. This page may be reproduced for classroom use only.

I Have Feelings!

LEARNING OBJECTIVES

■ Children will identify various emotions they feel in specific situations.

■ Children will begin to display acceptable behavior for expressing various emotions.

■ Children will cope with situations by exhibiting problem solving.

Planned activities are important for increasing children's understanding of events and the emotions attached to those events; most important, however, is helping children express emotions as they occur. Children learn from being part of many types of situations and circumstances and by watching how teachers and other adults act and react.

Often, young children respond to the emotions and reactions of the adults around them (known as emotional referencing); their behavior may be influenced by your actions and even facial expressions. If you are calm and exude happiness, then children are also more likely to be calm and happy. If, however, you arrive in a bad mood and your face and actions indicate that you are mad at the world, then the children's behavior may reflect your attitude. Be honest with children while remaining professional. It is okay for them to see that you have emotional responses, but you should model emotional expressions in an appropriate way.

Each day is filled with events that elicit a range of feelings (happiness, sadness, surprise, anger, love) in both children and adults. These reactions can become learning experiences when adults take time to talk with children about their own feelings and the children's feelings. If you are frustrated or sad, this may provide an opportunity to show children how to use problem-solving skills to determine effective ways of dealing with emotions. Another opportunity for discussion occurs when children are expressing various emotions. When children are playing together and smiling, you might remark on how happy they look and encourage the children to express how they feel.

When children cry, they may be hurt, sad, angry, or afraid. Encourage them to talk about what happened that made them cry, and ask how they feel about what happened. All emotions and feelings are okay; they are part of who we are as individuals. Acknowledge children's emotions, and help them express feelings in appropriate ways.

Some children may not know why they feel a certain way or may not have words to describe their feelings. Participating in an activity or in play that allows "acting out" or other ways of expressing themselves may help children. You and other adults can then help them match words with feelings and assist them in strengthening their problem-solving skills.

VOCABULARY

afraid	emotions	happy	proud
angry	excited	lonely	sad
awesome	express	mad	scared
bored	fear	meltdown	surprised
choose	feeling down	nightmare	
disappointed	feelings	patience	
embarrassed	glad	persistence	

CREATING THE ENVIRONMENT

- Include a schedule that allows time for discussion and processing, as well as for exercise and play, as outlets for emotional expression. Model listening and acceptance so that children feel comfortable in expressing their feelings.

- Play music from various genres, and display artwork from numerous artists. Provide a range of music, musical instruments, art supplies, water, and sand to encourage self-expression and emotional awareness. These materials, as well as dolls, toy people, dress-up clothes, puppets, and familiar props, promote exploration of feelings through role play.

EVALUATION

- Do children talk about how they feel emotionally?

- Do children use acceptable words to identify feelings?

- Do children use problem-solving skills to reach acceptable solutions?

- During role play, can children work through feelings?

- Can children demonstrate their feelings with appropriate actions (for example, with a laugh, smile, or frown)?

CHILDREN'S ACTIVITIES

Look at Me

Distribute to each child a mirror that is easy and safe to handle. In small groups, ask the children to look at themselves in their mirrors. Encourage them to make many kinds of faces. Then give them directions to make a happy face, a very happy face, a sad face, a very sad face, a mad face, a very mad face, an afraid face, a very afraid face. After they make each face, ask a few children to describe what their faces looked like, specifically their mouths and eyes. Talk with the children about how looking at a person's face may help us know how that person is feeling, but it also helps to use words to tell how we are feeling.

MATERIALS

- an unbreakable hand mirror for each child

OTHER IDEAS

- Read *Feelings to Share from A to Z* by Todd and Peggy Snow. Help children understand that people have many various feelings and that everyone has emotions.

- Encourage children to make faces using playdough. Ask children to talk about the feeling each face is showing.

- Let children use paper sacks or paper plates to make a series of masks showing different feelings. Help them measure where the eyeholes should be cut so they can wear their masks safely. Encourage children to talk about the feelings their masks are showing.

- Invite children to use string to measure their smile. Once they have their smile length of string, tell them to cut the string and measure it with a ruler. Encourage children to compare the string lengths of their smiles. Repeat with a frown, a scowl, and other facial expressions.

How Does It Feel?

Explain to children that you are going to tell them about a few activities, and they should close their eyes and imagine doing that activity while you are talking. Encourage the children to get comfortable before beginning. Tell a short descriptive story beginning with a statement such as, "Imagine that you. . . ." Use topics that can cause a range of emotions, such as playing with puppies, eating ice cream, being outside on a dark night, losing a special blanket, getting lost in a store, having a fast ride on a merry-go-round, swinging high in a swing, running very fast for a long time, finding a favorite toy broken, or visiting someone they love and then going home. After each story, encourage a few children to describe how they felt. Support and accept differences in feelings that children express. Help children see that everyone does not feel the same about an activity. Some children may love to play with puppies, but others may not like to get licked or may be afraid of them.

MATERIALS
- none

OTHER IDEAS
- Play, sing, and dance to happy songs, such as "Glad as Glad Can Be" by Grenadilla, "Joy to the World" by the Root Radics, "Sitting on Top of the World" by Grenadilla, and "If You Are Happy" by Tickle Tune Typhoon. Help children make a list of words that are like happy (glad, elated, joyful, cheerful, and so on).

- Play, listen to, and sing songs about fear, such as these songs by Justin Roberts: "Thought It Was a Monster," "Maybe the Monster," "Taking Off My Training Wheels," "Sleepover-land," "Never Getting Lost," "The Backyard Super Kid," and "Giant-Sized Butterflies." Discuss the songs, and let children express their opinions and feelings about similar situations.

- Read, role-play, and discuss books about sad feelings, such as *Glad Monster, Sad Monster* by Ed Emberley and Anne Miranda, *The Very Lonely Firefly* by Eric Carle, *Knuffle Bunny: A Cautionary Tale* by Mo Willems, and *Let's Talk about Feeling Sad* by Joy Berry.

■ Read, role-play, and discuss books about grouchy or mad feelings, such as *The Grouchy Ladybug* by Eric Carle, *Alexander and the Terrible, Horrible, No Good, Very Bad Day* by Judith Viorst, *Llama Llama Mad at Mama* by Anna Dewdney, and *When Sophie Gets Angry—Really, Really Angry . . .* by Molly Bang.

Dancing with Your Feelings

Play music samples representing various genres (country, blues, jazz, classical, hip-hop, and so on). Select music with a variety of beats, words, and paces. Invite children to dance with you to each type of music. After each sample of music, ask children how they felt when they heard the music. Show respect for everyone's feelings, and help children understand differences in preferences and in emotional reaction. Make a video of the activity, and at a later time let children study facial expressions and body language for signs of feelings.

MATERIALS

- music, music player, a video camera, a video monitor

OTHER IDEAS

- Invite children to choose from the classroom or bring from home music that makes them feel happy and want to dance. Play the music for children to share with others, and talk about how it makes them feel. Repeat the activity using different music.

  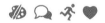

- Read and discuss *My Mama Sings* by Jeanne Whitehouse Peterson.

- Play a variety of music and invite children to play rhythm band instruments. Ask them how they felt during the activity. Remember that acceptable answers may include being bored.

- Lead children in making different sounds (groaning, sighing, mumbling, squealing, yawning, cooing, screaming, and so on). Encourage them to really get into the sound, making it several times. See if they can suggest other sounds for the group to make together. Ask how each sound made them feel.

Picture Feelings

Cover a large table with a paper tablecloth or large sheet of paper and secure it with tape. Divide the space and label areas as happy, sad, mad, afraid, bored, and so on. Encourage children to find and cut out photographs from magazines (or draw/paint their own) of things or activities that create feelings for them. Help children identify the appropriate space (based on their identified feelings) where their photos should be glued or taped onto the tablecloth. Encourage children to tell what is happening in their pictures and how they feel about it. See if children have ideas about what to do when they feel sad, mad, afraid, or bored. Help them think of acceptable ideas.

MATERIALS
- a paper tablecloth or large sheet of paper, tape, a marker, magazines, scissors, glue, and other art supplies requested by children

OTHER IDEAS

- Help children create a paper or electronic book in which to keep an image journal about their feelings. Encourage each child to make entries regularly, using cut-out photographs from magazines, drawings, paintings, photos, or other visual arts. Assist them with any captions or stories they want to add. Allow children to keep their journals private from other children, should they desire.

- Assist children in recording an individual video story about their various feelings. Talk with them about what they may want to include in the story. Prompt them with questions, if needed. Let children share their stories or keep them private from other children, if they wish.

- Invite children to select a picture from any book in the classroom that shows how they feel right now. Encourage children to explain why they picked the picture they did. Help them understand that it is okay if more than one child wants to pick the same picture or if they select a picture no one else did.

  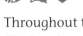

- Throughout the classroom space, display close-up facial shots reflecting a wide range of emotions. Include images on computer screen savers or slide shows.

Spinning Spider

Read and discuss with children *The Very Busy Spider* by Eric Carle. Point out that the spider was blown onto a fence and that it was probably surprised. Ask children to share good surprises they have had. Ask children to share any surprises they have had that they didn't like. Invite children to tell about what the spider did during the story. Help them see that the spider was determined and worked hard, even when others tried to get it to stop. Explain that sometimes when something is hard, it is important to keep working anyway. Ask children to share about a time they felt proud they could do something that required hard work. Reinforce the importance of working hard, and mention that when our feelings are strong, we sometimes have to work hard to find the best way to interact with others.

MATERIALS

■ *The Very Busy Spider* by Eric Carle

OTHER IDEAS

■ Read and discuss books in which characters are struggling with appropriate behavior, such as *My Mouth Is a Volcano!* by Julia Cook, *Cool Down and Work through Anger* by Cheri J. Meiners, *Hands Are Not for Hitting* by Martine Agassi, and *Words Are Not for Hurting* by Elizabeth Verdick. Help children identify appropriate alternatives for behavior as related to each book.

■ Read and discuss books to guide problem solving, such as *Don't Let the Pigeon Drive the Bus!* by Mo Willems, *I Did It, I'm Sorry* by Caralyn Buehner, *It Wasn't My Fault* by Helen Lester, and *Talk and Work It Out* by Cheri J. Meiners. Talk with children about how solving problems may be harder when we have strong feelings about something.

■ Play and listen to the words of "Take Time Out" by the Cat's Pajamas, "Stop, Think, Choose" and "Get Along" by Steve Couch, and "Pick Up the Pears" by Justin Roberts. Ask children what they think each song means. Help children identify ideas from the songs to help them deal with their emotions when they are mad, sad, or upset.

■ Play and listen to the words of "More Than Just a Minute" and "I Chalk" by Justin Roberts and "You've Got to Have Patience" by In the Nick of Time. Ask children if they find it hard to wait and what feelings they have when they need to wait. Help them identify acceptable things they can do while they wait and adults are busy (sing a song softly, draw in the air with their finger, stretch their bodies one part at a time, and so on). Let them practice some waiting activities for short periods.

Look at Them

Ask children to choose a partner, or group them into pairs. Have the partners in each group look at each other and make a happy face. Encourage partners to tell each other what their faces looked like. One at a time, suggest other faces to make (mad, sad, bored, scared), and discuss what they saw. Talk with the children about how everyone has feelings. Let them know that it is important to try and understand how others are feeling and to help them feel better when we can.

MATERIALS
- none

OTHER IDEAS

- Use a large nonbreakable mirror so the entire group can see themselves as they make faces that show various feelings. Encourage children to look at the faces made by others and compare them to their own.

- Have partners take photographs of each other while making a face to show emotion. Provide the photos electronically or in print form for children to look at and talk about.

- Play, listen to, and then sing songs that say others have emotions too, such as "Mama Is Sad" and "Meltdown" by Justin Roberts and "Just an Old Jalopy" by Cat's Pajamas. Talk about what each song means. Discuss with children how they may know if someone else is happy, sad, mad, or afraid.

- Play and listen to the words of "Making Silly Faces" by In the Nick of Time. Encourage children to think of various things they can do to help people feel better when they are sad, mad, or afraid.

FAMILY INFORMATION

I HAVE FEELINGS!

Children experience most of the same emotions adults experience: happiness, sadness, surprise, anger, and love. When children are playing together and smiling, remark on how happy they look, and encourage them to express how they feel.

When children cry, they may be feeling hurt, sad, angry, or afraid. Encourage your child to talk about what happened that made him or her cry, and ask how she or he feels about what happened. Often, just having you listen will help your child feel better.

Though we try, we cannot always accurately understand children's emotions. For example, a child who loses a loved one may feel confusion more than sadness. All emotions and feelings are okay; they are part of who we are as individuals.

INAPPROPRIATE ACTIONS

When children express anger or fright by hitting others or throwing toys, the behavior must be halted by firm and understanding intervention. After everyone calms down, talk about what happened that caused them to want to hit or throw. Help your child learn words for how she or he feels, and help your child find appropriate ways to show feelings. Learning to recognize different emotions takes time and practice.

MODEL APPROPRIATE BEHAVIOR

Children learn from many types of situations and circumstances and by watching how the adults in their lives act and react. Each day is filled with events that elicit the same feelings in both children and adults. These occasions can become learning experiences when you take time to talk with your child about your own feelings and your child's feelings.

FAMILY ACTIVITY

Glue this sheet to cardboard. Cut out the twenty-one individual dominoes. Turn all pieces facedown and mix them around. Leaving the pieces facedown, take turns drawing a domino from the mix until all dominoes have been chosen (if there is an even number of players, remove one domino). Players then turn their dominoes face up. The first player selects one of his or her dominoes to place in the center of the playing area. Players then take turns placing one of their dominoes to match the dominoes in the playing area. Matches can be a picture and an appropriate emotion, two of the same emotions, or two of the same pictures. If a player has no matches, the turn passes to the next player. The game is over when there are no more dominoes to match. As dominoes are matched, talk about the pictures, the emotions people feel, and what causes those feelings and emotions.

Key:

= happy

= scared

= mad

= sad

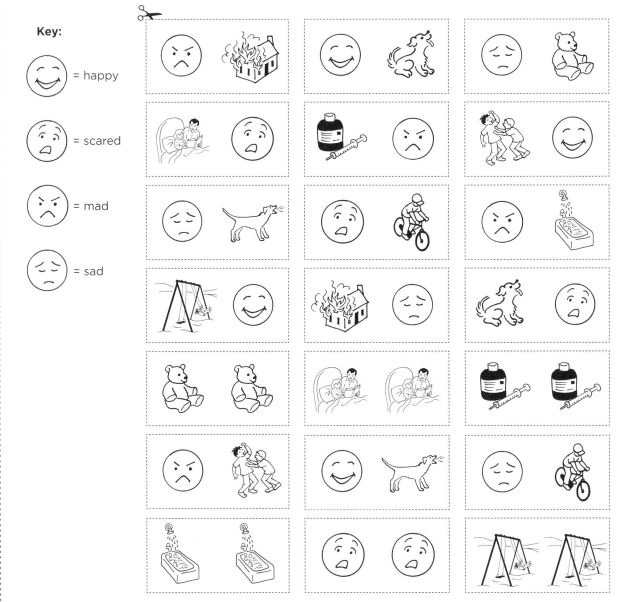

3

This Is My Family!

LEARNING OBJECTIVES

- Children will identify members of their family.
- Children will identify words associated with families.
- Children will express curiosity and acceptance of various family structures.

Children in your classroom will likely have a variety of family structures. They may live with two moms, two dads, a mom and a dad, one parent, an aunt or uncle, grandparents, older siblings, or foster parents. Some children will have experienced changes, such as divorce, that affect who resides in their home and how many homes they have. One child may have no brothers or sisters, while other children live with several siblings and perhaps other children (related or nonrelated). Help children to understand that every family is special and to respect differences.

Know whom the children in your program live with. If that is not possible, avoid using phrases that make assumptions, such as "take this home to your mother," since many children may be living with someone other than their mother. Instead, encourage children to take artwork, letters, and other materials home "to your family." Use books, pictures, songs, and words that include references to the many different adults who might be responsible for children.

Actively seek participation by every child's family; this is the best way to incorporate and include family structure, relationships, culture, traditions, and community issues relevant to each child's situation. When children encounter family styles or family activities different from their own, encourage acceptance and use reassuring words and phrases so children feel comfortable about their own family and other families.

Always keep family information confidential, whether it is shared by children in the classroom or provided by family members. Be sure to keep current records regarding emergency contacts for each child and any special help a child may need.

VOCABULARY

aunt	father	mother	sister
brother	few	pa	title
celebration	grandparent	pop	tradition
census	mama	relationship	uncle
cousin	many	relative	
dad	member	reunion	
daddy	mommy	ritual	

CREATING THE ENVIRONMENT

- Include books, pictures, and music representing every kind of family in your classroom and community.

- Make the classroom a welcome place for the children's family members by providing bulletin board displays, mailboxes, and a lending library especially for adults.

- Solicit ideas from all families regarding classroom visitors, family events, field trips, and activities so that the interests of a variety of families will be represented.

EVALUATION

- Do children act out a variety of family roles during play?

- Do children talk about their families and ask about other families during conversation?

- Do children use vocabulary associated with families?

- Can children identify individuals in their own families?

- Can children recognize and show respect for various family structures?

CHILDREN'S ACTIVITIES

Herd, Flock, and Pride

Show children a toy fish, and ask them if they know what a group of fish traveling together is called. Let them know it is a school. Show children a toy lion, ask if they know what a group of lions living together is called, and let them know it is a pride. Show children a toy monkey, and ask if they know what a group of monkeys together is called. Let them know it is a troop. Tell children that animals have communities and families that are sometimes like ours and sometimes are different. Introduce and read *Animal Families* by Lorrie Mack. Help children compare the animal families to their own.

MATERIALS

- a toy fish, a toy lion, a toy monkey, and *Animal Families* by Lorrie Mack (DK Publishing)

OTHER IDEAS

- Ask children to gather all of the toy animals from throughout the room. Once all animals are together in a designated spot, ask children to sort them into families any way they choose and to explain why they chose the family groups that they did. Help children understand that families of animals and families of people can look different in many ways.

- Read and discuss *And Tango Makes Three* by Justin Richardson and Peter Parnell, *Mister Seahorse* by Eric Carle, and *Animal Dads* by Sneed B. Collard III. Use these books to talk about the various ways to be a father.

- Read and discuss *Little Chick and Mommy Cat* by Marta Zafrilla. Use the book to introduce the idea of adoption in animal and human families.

- Ask children to share about any pets they have in their families. Read books about pets being part of the family, such as *Family Pets* by Lola M. Schaefer, *The Perfect Pet* by Margie Palatini, and *Pet Show!* by Ezra Jack Keats.

Taking a Census

Talk briefly about what a census is, how it is conducted, and why it is important. Involve each child in making a census booklet by stapling several pieces of blank paper together. For safety reasons, have them place tape over the staples. Children should create a title page for their booklet and include their name as author. Help children draw all of the people and pets who live with them. Be sensitive about the living situations of children, recognizing that some may have more than one household where they live and others may be homeless and live in shelters or cars. Focus on whom they live with rather than where they sleep. Once their drawings are complete, help the children label their family members and pets. Encourage children to share their booklets with each other so they can see the various kinds of families. Help children be respectful and help them understand family structures different from their own.

MATERIALS

- blank paper, markers, crayons, colored pencils, a stapler, and tape

OTHER IDEAS

- Create a census chart with each child's name down the left side and family member titles (Ma, Sister, Uncle, Baby) across the top. Be sure to include all family member titles represented in the children's families. Look at each child's census booklet and help each of them enter the correct numbers on the class chart to reflect their family. Remember that children may have more than one grandmother or mother, so using numbers rather than a check mark may more accurately reflect the families. Add each category, and talk with children about the totals for the class.

- Play and sing songs related to family, including "The Family Song" by Grenadilla, "How Many People in a Family" by the Cat's Pajamas, and "How Many People" by John McCutcheon.

- Read and discuss a variety of books about family, including *The Family Book* by Todd Parr, *All Kinds of Families!* by Mary Ann Hoberman, *Families* by Ann Morris, *A Tale of Two Daddies* by Vanita Oelschlager, and *Asha's Mums* by Rosamund Elwin and Michele Paulse.

■ Help each child count the people they live with and establish a total, including themselves. Instruct each child to gather one tabletop block for each person represented in her household and place a block on each picture or name in her census booklet. Ask children to return the blocks and repeat the activity using other toys.

Family Traditions Slide Show

To create a slide show representing all families of the children enrolled, ask families to contribute electronic close-up photographs of people and items (park frequently visited, vacation spot visited often, table decoration for holiday, jewelry handed down through generations, family crest, celebration symbols) that represent their traditions. Alternatively ask families to provide printed photos and items for you to photograph and return. Compile digital photos using presentation software, such as PowerPoint, or a photo-sharing service, such as Adobe Photoshop Express. Review the photos with each child, and assist him in selecting an order for his slides. Encourage children to dictate a caption for you to add for each photo. Help children create invitations for families to come and view the class Family Traditions Slide Show. As each child's slides are shown, allow the child to provide narration regarding the pictures or simply stand close to the screen.

MATERIALS
- photos contributed by families, a digital camera, presentation or photo-sharing software, a computer, and a screen and projector

OTHER IDEAS
- Assist each child in creating a song about the photographs contributed by his family for the slide show. Record the child singing the song, and play it with the slides, or allow children to sing the song live during the presentation for family members.

- Video children holding and talking about each of the photographs of family members and traditional items contributed by their family for a slide show. Provide copies of each individual child's video to his family.

- Play and sing the song "Tradition" by Topol. Discuss what the word *tradition* means.

- Read *The Lotus Seed* by Sherry Garland and *The Rag Coat* by Lauren Mills. Discuss family traditions and history with the children.

Puzzles, Puppets, and Playthings

Ask families to provide electronic or printed family photos for you to duplicate for use in activities. Return printed photos unharmed. Alternatively, take family photos during home visits or family events at the program. Make multiple photocopies of the photographs. Establish a place for each child's family photocopies, and let them use the photocopies for the following and other activities:

1. Attach a photocopy to cardboard, and cut it into puzzle pieces.

2. Create a hand puppet by cutting out family members' faces and other body parts and gluing them to a paper bag or an old sock.

3. Using Styrofoam, folded cardboard, or other free-standing material, assist children in attaching cutouts of family members to use as dollhouse figures or table toys.

4. Using two copies of the identical family photo, cut one copy in horizontal strips and the other in vertical strips. Weave the strips together to create the total picture again.

MATERIALS

- photocopies of family photos, cardboard, glue, scissors, paper bags, old socks, Styrofoam, and tape

OTHER IDEAS

- Use photocopies of the children and their families to mark their spaces, such as cubbies or coat hooks.

- Choose a family member's photo for each child, and enlarge it to make a mask.

- Let children choose a family photograph cut from a magazine to create stories or songs about the family.

- Involve children in using the copy machine to make duplicates of their family photos.

Family Relationships

Ask children to tell you what they call their father, mother, sister, brother, grandfather, grandmother, aunt, uncle, and any other relatives. As you identify titles used for father (Daddy, Dad, Pop, Pa), write each one down on a strip of paper. Repeat the process for all other family titles. Put strips of paper in a container. At a later time, remind children about the strips of paper you wrote family member titles on, and ask each child to take turns picking a slip of paper from the container. Read each slip of paper as it is selected, and help the children sort the strips into family categories, such as father or grandmother. Talk about how each family uses their own titles, some similar to and some different from other families. Include titles from languages representing the children enrolled. Extend this activity into the home by suggesting that children ask adults in their family what terms they use for their mother, father, and other family members.

MATERIALS
- a marker, strips of paper, and a container

OTHER IDEAS

- Play, sing, and discuss the song "Family Tree" by Tom Chapin.

- Read and discuss *The Relatives Came* by Cynthia Rylant.

- Invite children to cut multiple construction paper or cloth squares, all the same size. Encourage children to glue an individual picture of each family member on each square, and help them write the family title they use for each person. Let children arrange their squares into a quilt pattern. Guide them in punching holes on the sides of all squares where they will connect with another square. Provide yarn for them to lace their squares together. Take digital photos of each quilt, and display the photos in the classroom in a book, on a bulletin board, or on the computer.

- Ask the children who you are. Explain that to them you are their teacher, named _____, but you have other titles too. Show them photos of others who may call you something different, such as mother/father, sister/brother, daughter/son, aunt/uncle, niece/nephew, and any other relevant relationships. Help each child identify the different relationship titles they have, such as sister to ____, daughter of ____, and niece of ____. Explain that one person may have many different titles or names. Make a class chart with children's names down the side and relationship titles across the top. Help children make marks in the appropriate space to represent the relationship titles they have. Include some relationship titles that none of them will be able to mark, such as grandfather and grandmother.

Family Fun

Play "Three Days" by Justin Roberts, and listen to the words. Show children several photographs or drawings of diverse families (real or created for this activity) engaged in fun pastimes (hiking, swimming, playing a board game, reading, and so on). Ask the children if they and their family have ever taken part in any of the activities shown and what they thought about them. Invite children to share about other fun activities they have done with their families. Remind children that families may do some of the same fun things as other families, or they may do other things for fun.

MATERIALS

- photographs or drawings of several families (each with a different family composition) engaged in various fun activities

OTHER IDEAS

- Survey each child's family to obtain examples of what they do for fun. Focus on typical kinds of activities, such as going to the park, watching movies, swimming, hiking, playing board games, or singing songs. Compile a chart showing each child's name on the side and pictures of fun activities across the top. Mark each area based on the family survey. Share the results with the children, pointing out the similarities and differences.

- Show the children examples of simple scrapbooks, and explain that some people make scrapbooks as a way to remember and think about fun times. Provide materials and encourage children to make a scrapbook about their family's fun. Invite families to assist their child in this activity.

- Invite families of children enrolled and others from the program and the community to come and share with children what their families do for fun. Encourage them to bring props (hiking boots, a swim cap, rappelling ropes, and so on) to show children as they share.

- Collect brochures of local recreational spots (state parks, museums, zoos, and so on) in your community. Include some that are free and others that may have a fee. Show them to the children, and read selected parts. Encourage them to talk about any of the places they and their families have visited. Better yet, use the brochures to involve the children in selecting and planning an outing, and invite all families to join in the fun.

FAMILY INFORMATION

THIS IS MY FAMILY!

There are many different family structures. Children may live with two parents, one parent, an aunt, grandparents, or foster parents. A child may be an "only" or may have several brothers or sisters. Every family is special in its own way.

All children need a sense of belonging and the security of a family. Family structures sometimes change due to death, divorce, marriage, or the addition of a brother or sister. If family change is part of your child's life, discuss both it and its impact with her or him so that changes will be less confusing and frightening.

FAMILY CONTACT INFORMATION

Your child's school must be able contact you in case of emergency. Give your home, cell, and work phone numbers to your child's teacher or school office worker. If any of these numbers change, be sure to update your child's emergency contact file.

Teachers also need to know whom to call if they cannot reach you. This may be a family member, a neighbor, or a friend. If there are certain people who should never pick up your child, be sure the school knows this too.

Remember that schools must keep all family information confidential.

FAMILY ACTIVITY

Copy or trace the apples and leaves below (or draw your own), and help your child cut out and add the names (or pictures) of family members before attaching the apples/leaves to your family tree. Discuss the relationships of family members. Consider adding the dogs, cats, and other "members" of the family!

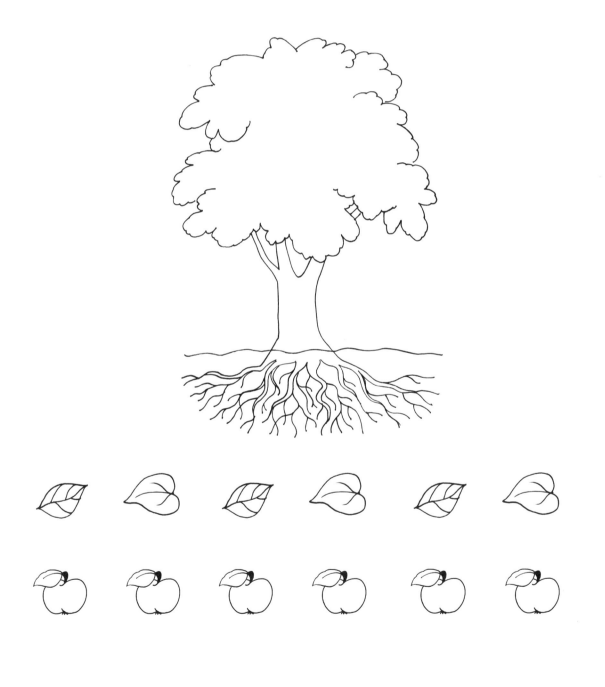

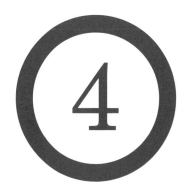

My Friends and Me!

LEARNING OBJECTIVES

- Children will identify individuals who are their friends and ways they play together.
- Children will practice courteous behavior and words with other children and adults, showing respect.
- Children will recognize and show respect for differences in clothing styles.

Children's views of the world and their understanding of people in their community are based on their experiences. Some young children live in close stable communities, surrounded by families who resemble their families and who have similar cultural and religious beliefs. Other children are exposed to a variety of family structures and people of various races, ethnic groups, and cultures. Children may also be exposed to differences in clothing, hairstyles, and physical abilities.

Sometimes a child's first experience with someone of a race, culture, or ability other their own may be in preschool or kindergarten. Children are curious and generally accept differences in other children, especially if teachers and other adults model respect for and acceptance of others. For example, clothing choices may be related to family, cultural, or religious background. Clothing is a significant part of individual and group identification. Learn the correct terminology for and the significance of special clothing used by the families in your classroom and community. As long as children's safety or health is not at risk be accepting of family choices.

You may want to refer to *Children Just Like Me: Celebrations!* by Barnabas and Anabel Kindersley, which provides pictures and information about clothing from around the world. Learning the differences between clothes worn for celebration and those worn for daily living will help with avoiding stereotyping. Ann Morris provides examples of clothing diversity in her book *Hats, Hats, Hats*. She shows that covering one's head can be for decoration, respect, worship, or safety. Hard hats, sun hats, and firefighter hats are among the many examples included.

Children often experience feelings of friendliness before they have words to describe or encourage a friendship. When children first join a group or class, they may revert to the initial stages of play and simply play alongside another. Even as children begin to interact more, they still need opportunities to play alone, as well as alongside and with others.

Friendships for young children may come and go quickly based on the situation at the moment. Encourage children to respect others as they begin to form friendships. Tell them that one way to show respect is by behaving courteously. Guiding children to use words such as "please," "thank you," "you're welcome," "excuse me," and "I'm sorry" helps them learn to respect other people.

As you model and guide the use of respectful language and behavior, make sure your expectations for children are culturally and developmentally appropriate. Stop behaviors that are hurtful, discriminatory, or unfair to others, and explain why those behaviors hurt people.

VOCABULARY

alike	courteous	imaginary	polite
apologize	different	invite	problem
bully	friend	join	respectful
cheerful	friendship	listen	share
compliment	generous	lonely	take turns
cooperate	helpful	manners	trade

CREATING THE ENVIRONMENT

- Include time each day for children to play together and alone. Allow some freedom for children to sit by whom and where they want, such as during mealtime or group activities.

- Make available outdoor materials and equipment to promote socialization, such as a double slide, a trike with a double seat, and a playhouse. Indoors have children use art and woodworking materials to make items for friends. Promote activities that include and encourage communication and cooperation between children.

■ In your interest centers, include clothing items worn by the culture and ethnic groups of children's families and of people in the local community, books and music representing these cultures, and dolls that look like the children in your classroom and the people in the community.

EVALUATION

■ Do children play with others peacefully?

■ Do children use courtesy words?

■ Do children recognize showing respect for differences in others?

■ Do children show a preference for some clothing styles yet accept people who have other preferences?

■ Can children discuss who their friends are?

CHILDREN'S ACTIVITIES

Playing with Friends

Encourage children to contribute to a classroom mural about playing with friends. Children can draw or paint pictures of toys they and their friends like to play with or activities they like to do together. Children can add pictures found in magazines of friends sharing with each other, helping each other, or showing affection. Encourage children to talk about their contributions to the mural and what it means to be a friend.

MATERIALS

- a large sheet of paper attached to a wall or tabletop, markers, crayons, colored pencils, and paint

OTHER IDEAS

- Read *Friends* by Helme Heine. Encourage children to compare what they do with their friends to the activities of the friends in this book.

- Play "Cartwheels & Somersaults" by Justin Roberts and move to the music and listen to the words. Invite the children to talk about what the friends in the song did together, and ask what they do for fun with their friends.

- Take photographs of children playing together inside and outside. Select and print photos showing every child engaged with another. Provide each child with his photo, and invite him to tell about what he was doing with his friend. Involve each child in gluing her photo to cardboard, laminating it if possible, and cutting it into puzzle pieces. Encourage children to work their puzzles with their friends in the picture.

  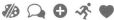

- Take photographs of groups of children during various parts of the day. Select and print photos, ensuring that all children are represented. Provide each child with two identical photos, and help the children glue each photo to cardboard and laminate them if possible. Help children use a ruler to measure and draw equal squares on the photos and then cut on the lines. Show children how to turn all pieces from both photos picture-side down to play a memory game. Provide a container, and leave the memory game in the table toys interest area.

Tug-of-War

Provide natural manila rope, and involve children in finding the halfway point on the rope. Tie a piece of cloth at the halfway point. Teach children how to play tug-of-war, beginning with small groups. After the game, talk with children about how friends need to work together, and ask if they worked together in tug-of-war. Help them see that each team worked together to try and pull the red cloth to their side, but each team also worked (pulled) against the other team (friends). Ask how they felt about the game. Explain that when everyone agrees to the game, pulling can be fun, but we all need to know how to work together too. Let them know that when people work together, it is called cooperation.

MATERIALS

- natural manila rope (not synthetic rope, especially not nylon)

OTHER IDEAS

- Instruct pairs of children to stand face-to-face with the palms of their hands touching. Ask the children to work together in moving toward one side five steps and then back again. Show children how to step one foot and slide the other to meet it, so that they are walking sideways. Encourage each pair to find other ways to walk together cooperatively.

- Provide a large ball, and involve two or more children in moving it from one place to another together. Help children identify as many ways as possible to move the ball together.

- Hold three-legged sack (or pillowcase) walks and runs, not races with winners and losers. Challenge pairs to set their own goals and run the distance agreed upon. Point out that the children worked together if they were successful in walking or running when each had one leg in the sack.

- Teach children rhythm clapping games to do in pairs or larger groups. Make up patterns, or use traditional games and songs. Encourage children to practice in pairs, and slowly incorporate more people as they become more skillful. Talk with them about the importance of watching their partner and working together for the game to be successful.

With a Little Help

Play, sing, and dance to the song "With a Little Help from My Friends" by the Beatles. Ask the children what they think the song means. Tell them that being helpful is one of the things friends do for each other. Encourage children to generate a list of ways friends can help each other, and write down all of their ideas so you can refer to them later. End the activity by letting children know that helping is one of the ways to be a good friend.

MATERIALS

- "With a Little Help from My Friends" by the Beatles, a music player, chart paper, and a marker

OTHER IDEAS

- Introduce the concept of friendship bracelets, and show children examples or pictures of various bracelets. Talk about the patterns and how each bracelet is a different style. Provide a variety of materials (yarn, beads, and so on) and general suggestions for creating bracelets for friends. Have some bracelets made by the teachers to share with children who have never received a friendship bracelet. Remind children that sharing and giving are ways to be a good friend.

- Let children know you are going to play a listening game. Explain that everyone will close their eyes, hold out their hands, and listen. Tell them you will put a ball in one child's hands. The person with the ball should then loudly say, "I have the

ball," and everyone will guess who has it. Ask children to open their eyes between the times the ball is given to a child. After the game, talk about how listening is an important way to be a good friend.

- Read and discuss *"I Have a Little Problem," Said the Bear* by Heinz Janisch. Talk with children about how friends listen and help each other with problems. See if children can tell you about a time when a friend listened to them or when they listened to a friend.

- Read and discuss in small groups *How to Be a Friend* by Laurie Krasny Brown and Marc Brown.

Row, Row, Row Your Boat

Teach the children the song "Row, Row, Row Your Boat," and show them the motion for rowing oars. Introduce the concept of singing in rounds, and demonstrate with another adult how that is done. Divide children into two groups, explaining that each group should begin singing the song when you point to them. Try the rounds with more groups after using two has been successful. After singing, talk with children about how it is sometimes harder to begin playing with a friend than it is to begin singing with them. Ask what ideas they have about how to get someone to play with them. Help them see that they can invite someone to play or they can ask to join in play. Give them examples of words they can use, and let them practice.

MATERIALS
- none

OTHER IDEAS

- Play, dance to, and listen to the words of "C'mon C'mon" by Grenadilla. Remind children that friends invite other friends to play with them.

- Teach children traditional songs, like "Playmate, Come Out and Play with Me" and "The More We Get Together." Let children know that they can talk or sing to invite friends to play with them.

- Read and discuss *Join In and Play* by Cheri J. Meiners. Role-play with children to help them practice their joining-in play skills.

- Read *Manners* by Aliki or another book about manners. Play, listen to, and dance to "Great Big Sun" by Justin Roberts. Let children know that friends are polite and use good manners. Ask a series of "What would be the polite thing to say if . . . ?" questions to give children an opportunity to practice using good manners.

Imaginary Friends

Play, sing, and dance to "Our Imaginary Rhino" by Justin Roberts. Ask children what they know about imaginary friends, and encourage them to share stories. Guide children in creating imaginary friends by asking them to decide if their friend is a boy or a girl, by helping them describe their friend's physical characteristics, and by encouraging them to give their friend a name. Demonstrate for children how to introduce someone, and invite them to introduce their imaginary friends to the group.

MATERIALS

- "Our Imaginary Rhino" by Justin Roberts, a music player

OTHER IDEAS

- Read and discuss stories about being lonely and making friends, such as *Biff, the Lonely Great White Shark* by Maria Gilleard, *The Very Lonely Firefly* by Eric Carle, and *The Lonely Little Monster* by Andi Green. Talk with the children about what being lonely means, encourage them to share any stories about being lonely, and reassure children that everyone feels lonely sometimes.

- Read *A Rainbow of Friends* by P. K. Hallinan and *All Kinds of Friends, Even Green!* by Ellen B. Senisi. Talk about how each person is an individual with features, such as black hair, that many other people also have. Compare the eye color, hairstyle, skin color, and clothing style that children wear as examples of similarities and differences. Help children see that similarity does not equal good and difference does not mean bad.

- Read and discuss books that show how children can feel friendship with a tree, a pet, or other unconventional friends. Book examples include *The Giving Tree* by Shel Silverstein and *Taking a Bath with the Dog and Other Things That Make Me Happy* by Scott Menchin.

- Teach children the song "Make New Friends, but Keep the Old," and read *Rainbow Fish to the Rescue!* by Marcus Pfister. Encourage children to identify friends they have had for a long time and ways to make new friends.

No Bullies Allowed

Play and listen to the words of "Billy the Bully" by Justin Roberts. Ask children what they think about the song. Read *Lucy and the Bully* by Claire Alexander. Without identifying anyone specifically, ask children what they know about bullies. Help children understand that acting like a bully is inappropriate and so is name-calling. Encourage them to let an adult know if they have trouble with someone so the adult can help.

MATERIALS

- "Billy the Bully" by Justin Roberts, a music player, and *Lucy and the Bully* by Claire Alexander

OTHER IDEAS

- Read *How to Lose All Your Friends* by Nancy Carlson. Help children identify things they should do if they want to keep their friends and make new ones.

- Encourage children to show you everything they can do with their hands that will not hurt themselves, hurt others, or damage property. Read and talk about *Hands Are Not for Hitting* by Martine Agassi from the Best Behavior Series. Consider reading other books from the series, such as *Teeth Are Not for Biting* and *Feet Are Not for Kicking.*

- Read and discuss *Best Best Friends* by Margaret Chodos-Irvine. Let the children act out the book, using the solution the author did and then creating other solutions of their own. Help children understand that even best friends have fights, but it is important to try and work things out.

- Play, dance to, and sing "Best Friend" by Justin Roberts. Explain that it sometimes takes talking and problem solving to stay best friends, even when you have a lot of fun together. Read and discuss *Talk and Work It Out* by Cheri J. Meiners.

FAMILY INFORMATION

MY FRIENDS AND ME!

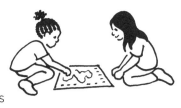

Some children are outgoing and make friends easily. Other children are more comfortable by themselves or with just one or two other children. Your child may have a best friend or two, or friends he or she enjoys playing with the most. Talk with your child about being a friend, and ask who her or his friends are.

It is not uncommon for children to say, "No one likes me." If your child says this, he or she likely feels that way at the moment. Try to find out why. It could be that another child has hurt your child's feelings. Or it might be that your child is not sure how to talk or play with other children yet. When these types of situations occur, discuss how to be a friend to others. It is easier to have friends when you are being a friend.

RESPECT FOR FRIENDS AND STRANGERS

Encourage your child to respect others as she or he begins to form friendships. Tell your child that one way to show respect is by behaving courteously. Guiding children to use words such as "please," "thank you," "you're welcome," "excuse me," and "I'm sorry" helps them learn to respect other people.

From Social and Emotional Well-Being by Connie Jo Smith, Charlotte M. Hendricks, and Becky S. Bennett,
© 2014. Published by Redleaf Press, www.redleafpress.org. This page may be reproduced for classroom use only.

FAMILY ACTIVITY

Attach the following photograph to cardboard or an empty cereal box. Cut out the pieces. As you help your child work the puzzle, discuss which activities people he or she knows like to do for fun and how we can have many friends who like to do different things than we do. Talk about some of the differences, and ask how your child's friends are the same as and different from her or him.

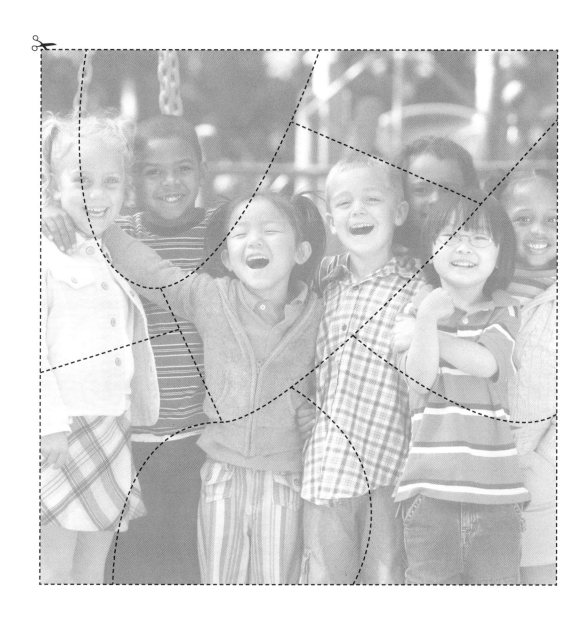

From *Social and Emotional Well-Being* by Connie Jo Smith, Charlotte M. Hendricks, and Becky S. Bennett, © 2014. Published by Redleaf Press, www.redleafpress.org. This page may be reproduced for classroom use only.

⑤

My World Is Changing

LEARNING OBJECTIVES

- Children will recognize changes in their school, home, and natural environment (for example, new students, stages of insect growth, seasonal plant changes, a new pet, and an additional family member).
- Children will state ways to prepare for changes in weather (for example, having a raincoat or sunglasses).
- Children will try new experiences (for example, play a new game, use a different piece of playground equipment, taste an unfamiliar food).

Children of all ages need consistency in their lives. They need to know above all that they are loved and that someone will take care of them. They develop self-esteem and feelings of security through attachments to nurturing adults, daily routines, even favorite toys or blankets that hold special places in their lives. Security through consistency helps children adapt to change when it occurs.

There are many positive changes in children's lives—change to a new classroom or teacher, new toys and games to play with, and meeting new friends. Some changes may be more challenging and even traumatic for children: change in their families or homes may occur from fire or weather-related events or from loss of a parent or family member through divorce or death; they may acquire a new parent or siblings through blended families; or friends or a much-loved pet may be left behind if they move to a new home or community.

Some children seem to adapt to changes easily, whereas others take more time. But remember, all children need consistency. If changes occur in the home or family, it becomes even more important for children to have consistent, nurturing adults at school. Continue with familiar routines for eating, playtime, circle time, naptime, and other regularly scheduled activities.

Talk with children about changes that are expected, such as moving to a new classroom or getting a new teacher. Children respond to adult emotions and actions, so convey a positive approach to change. Let them know that they will still have consistency, love, and security in important areas of their lives.

VOCABULARY

adapt	death	marriage	sleepover
adjust	divorce	metamorphosis	try
baby	first	moving	unknown
caterpillar	grow	new	weight
chameleon	height	pupa	
change	larva	relocating	
cocoon	leap	sand castle	

CREATING THE ENVIRONMENT

- Provide extra outerwear (raincoats, galoshes, umbrellas) as needed for local weather conditions.

- To help children from various family configurations feel welcomed, display photographs of children and their families. Include photos to represent dual homes, blended families, and family additions (new baby, marriage).

- Document and display the enrolled children's changes and progression through the year with growth charts, representations of developing skills, and photographs. Provide a place for children in the program to post photographs of themselves and their family members.

- Place familiar objects in unusual places throughout the classroom and playground for children to notice, and discuss the change. For example, hang an umbrella from the ceiling low enough that children need to walk around or go under it, put a nonpoisonous flowering plant on the floor in a walkway, and place a kitchen pot full of water in the middle of the trike path.

EVALUATION

- Do children talk about changes in weather or in nature?

- During pretend play, do children role-play changes they have experienced or heard about (for example, taking care of a new baby or a new pet)?

■ Do children express thoughts or feelings about changes in their environment (for example, a different home, a sick family member, or new clothes)?

■ Are children open to changes in the classroom and on the playground, such as new toys or books?

■ Do children willingly try new experiences?

CHILDREN'S ACTIVITIES

Weather Floor Memory Game

Give each child one of your twenty weather-related photographs, and place any extras face up in the masking tape frames on the floor. Take turns having children describe the photograph they are holding. At the end of each turn, involve children in finding the photograph that is just like the one described. Once all matches have been found, ask children to help you place photographs facedown in the tape frames. Introduce the game of memory, and explain the rules. Let them know they will be taking turns picking two photos to turn over to see if they are alike. If the photos match, they go into a matched pile. If they do not match, they are turned back over for the next person's turn. After the game, talk about how the weather changes and that we cannot stop it from changing, but we can sometimes get ready for the change. Ask children what we do to get ready if it is going to rain (for example, wearing boots or carrying an umbrella). Ask children what we do to get ready for the sun (sunscreen, umbrella or tent or shade tree, water play, and so on). Ask children about other local weather conditions.

MATERIALS
- two copies of ten distinctively different weather-related photos (from the Internet, calendars, and so on), each 8½ by 11 inches and laminated for endurance, and masking tape placed on the floor to indicate the twenty frames where the photographs go

OTHER IDEAS
- Read and talk about *Wings of Change* by Franklin Hill. Add a butterfly garden to the classroom, and study the four stages (egg, larva, pupa, adult) of butterfly metamorphosis. Talk about the changes the butterfly goes through.

- Add kits to raise and observe changes in ladybugs, frogs, praying mantises, sea monkeys, or earthworms. Help

children track the changes and compare them to other familiar changes.

- Read and discuss books about change in nature, such as *The Mixed-Up Chameleon* by Eric Carle. Talk about the importance of being one's self, but also share a few facts about chameleons. Let children know that some chameleons can change colors and do so to communicate their mood. Some change colors to camouflage for safety.

- Play and listen to the words of "Sand-castle" by Justin Roberts. Encourage children to build a sand castle and then wash it away in waves using a water hose or a bucket of water. Talk about how they changed the sand into the castle and then how the water changed the sand again. Invite children to share how they felt about the sand activity.

Once a Little Baby

Show children some clothes for a newborn baby. Tell them that they were all small enough to wear those clothes when they were babies, but they have grown a lot since then. Ask children what changes they have experienced since they were small enough to wear the baby clothes. Help them become aware of their physical changes, new skills, and interests. Encourage children to share what they like about growing and changing and what they do not like about it. Explain that we all continue to grow and change; even adults change the older they get.

MATERIALS

■ various newborn baby clothes

OTHER IDEAS

■ Read and discuss *Harry the Happy Caterpillar Grows: Helping Children Adjust to Change* by Cindy Jett. Talk about how the caterpillar grew and changed and how the children's bodies are growing and changing.

■ Play and listen to the words of "Apple Tree" by Justin Roberts. Assure children that they may not be as big as they want to be right now, but they will continue to grow and get bigger. Weigh and measure each child, and compare the data to their weight and height later in the year.

■ Play and listen to the words of "Old Pajamas" by Justin Roberts. Ask children if they have ever had some clothes or toys that they did not want to give up, even though they had outgrown them and were getting new ones. Acknowledge the feelings people have about the loss of things.

■ Read and discuss *Naked Mole Rat Gets Dressed* by Mo Willems. Ask children if they understand how Wilbur feels about clothes and how they can help him feel funny, fancy, or cool. Encourage children to share how various clothes make them feel.

Give It a Try

Show children a bucket of rocks. Take one out, and tell the children about something new that you have tried. Then invite each child to take a rock and talk about something new he has tried. If a child has nothing new to share, help her find a fast and easy new thing to do, like making a funny face or a strange sound. Tell children that trying new things means a change from the old, and it can be scary for some. Let them know you are going to read a story about Lizzy being afraid. Read and discuss *When Lizzy Was Afraid of Trying New Things* by Inger Maier.

MATERIALS

- Bucket of rocks and *When Lizzy Was Afraid of Trying New Things* by Inger Maier

OTHER IDEAS

- Play, dance to, and listen to the words of "Sleepoverland" by Justin Roberts. Ask children if they have ever spent the night somewhere other than where they live, maybe with a friend, an aunt, or grandparents. Listen to stories they share, and let them know that even though it sometimes can be frightening, it also can be great fun to have a sleepover.

- Read and discuss *The Girl Who Never Made Mistakes* by Mark Pett and Gary Rubinstein or *Nobody's Perfect: A Story for Children about Perfectionism* by Ellen Flanagan Burns.

- Show children a set of training wheels, and ask if anyone knows what they are and why they are used. Play and listen to the words of "Taking Off My Training Wheels" by Justin Roberts. Talk with children about how the child in the song felt.

- Read and discuss *PEEP! A Little Book about Taking a Leap* by Maria van Lieshout.

Moving

Play and listen to the words of "Moving" by Justin Roberts. Let children know that sometimes when people move to a different home or a different town, it is called relocating. Ask children questions such as the following:

- Have you ever moved to a new home?

- Do you know anyone who has moved?

- What does a family do to get ready to move?

- What does a family have to pack?

- How does a family move their things?

- What is the best thing about moving to someplace new?

- What is the worst thing about moving to someplace new?

- How do families make friends when they move?

MATERIALS

- "Moving" by Justin Roberts, a music player

OTHER IDEAS

- Provide boxes, suitcases, luggage carts, and a wagon for children to role-play packing and moving or to use as props as they tell about a moving experience.

- Take a field trip to a moving company, or watch a video clip of movers working. Look at the trucks, lifts, and other tools that help make moving go smoothly.

- Read and talk about *Alexander, Who's Not (Do You Hear Me? I Mean It!) Going to Move* by Judith Viorst.

- Read *Amelia's Road* by Linda Jacobs Altman.

  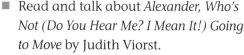

Changing Families

Read and discuss *Presto Change-O* by Audrey Wood. Tell children that the changes in families are not usually like the magical changes in *Presto Change-O*. Ask children what changes their family has had. Prompt children who you know have had some changes, like the addition of new family members. Acknowledge that some changes can be really hard at first, even if they are good ones.

MATERIALS

- *Presto Change-O* by Audrey Wood

OTHER IDEAS

- Using toy people, show children a family, and introduce each family member. Provide numerous other people and pet figures, and ask a child to change the family you introduced in some way by adding or taking away family members. Count with the children the number of family members before and after the change. Continue to let children make changes and describe the changes they choose to make. End the activity by giving each child access to figures to create a family of their own, which may or may not represent their actual family. Casually point out that families may change many times.

- Read and discuss books about new babies arriving, such as *Changes* by Anthony Browne, *Will There Be a Lap for Me?* by Dorothy Corey, *The New Baby at Your House* by Joanna Cole, and *Peter's Chair* by Ezra Jack Keats.

- Read and discuss books about blended families and marriages, such as *Do You Sing Twinkle?: A Story about Remarriage and New Family* by Sandra Levins, and *Jessica's Two Families: Helping Children Learn to Cope with Blended Households* by Lynne Hugo.

- Read and discuss books about separation and divorce, such as *Dinosaurs Divorce: A Guide for Changing Families* by Laurene Krasny Brown and Marc Brown, *Fred Stays with Me!* by Nancy Coffelt, and *My Family's Changing* by Pat Thomas.

Building Changes

Show *Changes, Changes* by Pat Hutchins, and ask children as you show each page of this picture book what they think is happening and how they think the characters feel. Point out that the characters in this book had many changes, but they found ways to make the changes work through problem solving and adapting. Build something with blocks, and then rearrange the same blocks to be something else. Engage each child in building something and then changing it.

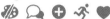

MATERIALS

- a copy of *Changes, Changes* by Pat Hutchins, and building blocks for each child

OTHER IDEAS

- Play and listen to the words of "Three Little Pigs" by Justin Roberts. Help children compare this song to the book *Changes, Changes* by Pat Hutchins.

- Read *Harold and the Purple Crayon*, 50th Anniversary Edition, by Crockett Johnson, and play "I Chalk" by Justin Roberts. Help children compare this book and song so they see that both characters were able to change their drawing as they needed to.

- Play and listen to the words of "Roller in the Coaster" by Justin Roberts and "The Way It Goes" by Grenadilla. Talk with children about what the songs mean. Help them understand the concept of going with the flow or bending with the wind.

- Teach children the words to both verses of "I'm a Little Teapot," and demonstrate how they can use one arm for a handle and one for a spout. Let them act it out while they sing. Then show children how to change which arm is the handle and which is the spout before singing and acting it out again. Help them see that the teapot was adaptable, a skill that is important for all people. Follow up by reading *I'm a Little Teapot* by Iza Trapani.

FAMILY INFORMATION

MY WORLD IS CHANGING

All children need love, nurturing, and consistency in their daily lives. They develop self-esteem and feelings of security through attachments to nurturing adults, daily routines, and even their favorite toy or blanket. By promoting feelings of security every day, you can help your child adapt to changes that occur in his or her life.

Some changes are exciting and fun, such as entering school for the first time, anticipating a new baby brother or sister, or even changing bedroom and sleeping arrangements. But these same events may be more challenging for some children. Let children practice making small changes successfully, like trying a new flavor of ice cream or walking with you to the park using a different route.

BUILD TRUST

Talk with your child about expected changes, and assure your child that you will always have love and attention for her or him. Children respond to your emotions and actions, so present change in a positive way whenever possible. If practical, let children assist in preparing for change.

Help your child adapt to the big changes in his or her life by maintaining daily consistency as much as possible. Continue with familiar routines, such as family meals together, bedtime stories and hugs, and time for outdoor play. Let your child keep a favorite toy, blanket, or book—even if it is dirty and ragged!

Above all, let your child know that you love her or him and will be there to help through changes. Listen, show interest, and build trust through communication and actions with your young child. As you continue to build this relationship of communication and trust throughout the childhood and teenage years, you will help your child become a happy and well-adjusted young adult.

From *Social and Emotional Well-Being* by Connie Jo Smith, Charlotte M. Hendricks, and Becky S. Bennett, © 2014. Published by Redleaf Press, www.redleafpress.org. This page may be reproduced for classroom use only.

FAMILY ACTIVITY

Change is sometimes very hard for a young child, whether it is a new family member or a change in the family structure, a change from one school or day care to another, a change in friends, or a move to a new home. You may wish to cut out a set of the pictures below that best represents a current change in your child's life (or you and your child could draw your own pictures) and put one picture at the beginning of the maze and the other at the end. You may then wish to assist your child in finishing the maze while you talk with him or her about how best to "navigate" the current or upcoming change and about developing a plan for how she or he can help prepare for it.

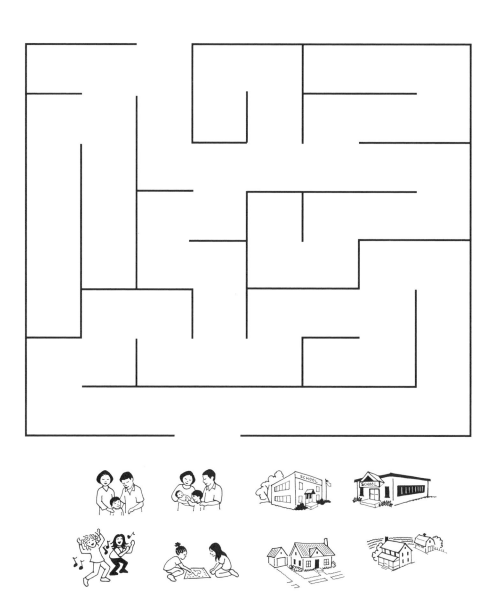

When Someone or Something Special to Me Dies

LEARNING OBJECTIVES

- Children will use terms related to death, dying, and ceremonies surrounding death.
- Children will communicate emotions and feelings related to death experiences.
- Children will recognize that death rituals are unique to each culture.

Even young children may experience situations and loss related to death—the death of a family member, a friend, or a much loved pet. Introduce this topic by giving examples of real experiences that teachers, children, or families have had, or use examples from nature. Since various religions, cultures, and families have different rituals and beliefs surrounding death, explore a variety of terms, rituals, and emotions so you do not inadvertently promote the ideas of any group over another.

Concentrate on gathering and providing information on the death customs of the cultures and families represented in your classroom. It is also helpful to include information from cultures not represented, thereby giving children a broader understanding as they interact with other people in their communities.

Provide ample opportunity for children to ask questions. Answer honestly, but if you do not have an answer, explain that you do not know, and involve children in research to find possible answers. You might also ask children what they think instead of trying to provide answers yourself. Facilitate discussion by reading books on the topic aloud, listening to music that deals with the topic, inviting guests to share information, allowing children to talk about their experiences in a group, and observing nature.

Children may not understand that the person or pet who has passed away will not return. Characters in cartoons, television programs, movies, and video games often are portrayed as dead or dying, yet they appear the next day or week in a new program. Young children may not comprehend that situations they view through media may not be real.

VOCABULARY

bury	deceased	headstone	tomb
cemetery	epitaph	hearse	tombstone
coffin	eulogy	mausoleum	visitation
cremate	extinct	memorial service	wake
crypt	feelings	monument	
dead	funeral	sorrow	
death certificate	grief	sympathy	

CREATING THE ENVIRONMENT

- Include books and music that connect with some aspect of death, or music that might be used during various death rituals. Provide materials in activity centers that promote role play of rituals or ceremonies.

- Help children see the processes involved and the connection between life and death by creating a space indoors or outdoors that is devoted to growing things. If space is not available, use nature walks, field trips, books, and video clips to explore the life cycle of various plants, trees, animals, and birds that can be found in your area.

- Be sensitive to children's fears and emotions related to situations and experiences. For example, a child who lost a family member or pet in a tornado or fire may be frightened by weather conditions or warning alarms. Help children understand and express such fears; work with family members to help children learn to cope with these situations.

EVALUATION

- Do children talk about someone or something dying and use related words?

- Are children role-playing about ceremonies or rituals related to death?

- Do children show respect for death rituals unfamiliar to them?

- As appropriate, do children express thoughts or feelings related to death (for example, of a pet, a plant, or a person)?

- In guided activities, do children participate in a death ritual (for example, the death of a goldfish or a plant)?

CHILDREN'S ACTIVITIES

Living or Not

Show children a display that includes living things and things that are not living or have died. Include at least one display item per child. Ask children if someone can explain what alive (or living) means. Clarify that when something is alive, it drinks, eats, grows, moves, and responds to what goes on around it. Read *What's Alive?* by Kathleen Weidner Zoehfeld. Invite children to sort the items into living and not living groups. If they have trouble deciding, help them by asking questions, for example, "Do you think it grows?" Point out that the bug used to be alive and grew, but now it is no longer living. Let them know that we call it dead or deceased when something or someone was alive but is not alive any longer.

MATERIALS

- living things (plants, a fish, an earthworm, a child), things not living or that have died (rocks, a plastic toy, a cloth doll, a stainless steel spoon, dead bugs), and *What's Alive?* by Kathleen Weidner Zoehfeld

OTHER IDEAS

- Play "Safari" by Eek-A-Mouse. Explain to children that a safari is a land trip to see animals that are free in their natural habitat, unlike a zoo. Tell them that some people go on a safari to hunt (and kill) animals but most go to watch and take photographs.

- Go on a playground safari to look for things that are dead and things that are alive. Encourage children to look up in the sky and to examine the ground closely. Provide magnifying glasses, binoculars, and cameras. Discuss with children their findings.

- Tell children that living people and animals breathe. Show children how to put their hands close to their nostrils to feel their breath when they exhale. Let children put their hands near the nostrils of a classroom doll to feel that no air is being exhaled. Show them how to hold their breath, and let them practice. Explain that just holding their breath does not make them dead.

- Read *Epossumondas Plays Possum* by Coleen Salley. Explain to children that playing possum means acting like you are dead, but when you act like you are dead, you are still alive. Invite the children to play possum.

What Happens When It Dies?

Have children gather fallen and dead leaves and twigs, dead bugs, and dead plants to bring into the classroom. Use gloves, a cup, or tweezers to scoop up dead bugs. Set up in the classroom an observation space for all the leaves, twigs, bugs, and plants. Let children be responsible for designing labels that describe and date each item, either with words or drawings. Encourage children to observe over the course of time what happens to each item. Their observations can be recorded using a book, chart, drawing, photograph, or video, with assistance from the teacher as needed.

MATERIALS

- leaves, twigs, dead bugs, dead plants; container(s) for dead items; gloves, or a cup, or tweezers; labels, markers, and observation recording supplies (blank paper, pencils, a video camera, a still camera)

OTHER IDEAS

- Place a vegetable in a clear resealable bag or container with a lid. Let children monitor what happens to the vegetable and compare the process to the fallen and dead leaves and twigs, dead bugs, and dead plants. Help children understand that the vegetable was once alive and growing on a plant.

- Read and discuss *The Fall of Freddie the Leaf: A Story of Life for All Ages*, 20th Anniversary Edition, by Leo Buscaglia.

- Read and discuss selected pages from *When Dinosaurs Die: A Guide to Understanding Death* by Laurie Krasny Brown and Marc Brown. To follow up, make the book available for children to look at, and let them ask questions.

- Introduce an ant farm for children to observe. Encourage children to watch and discuss the many jobs the ants do, including moving any dead ants away from their living area.

Remembering the Good Things

This activity can be used at any time but may be most useful when a child in the classroom experiences the death of a pet, a friend, or a relative. Invite children to bring photos or drawings of someone or some creature they knew who died. Ask each child who brings a picture to display it in a special spot set aside for this activity and to show it to friends throughout the day. Introduce the term *eulogy*, and explain that a eulogy is a story about someone who has died. Encourage children to share something about a particular person, animal, or plant that died.

MATERIALS
- a space to display photos or drawings

OTHER IDEAS

- Read *Grandma's Scrapbook* by Josephine Nobisso. Talk with the children about keepsakes and memories.

- Play "The Letter" by Holly Near. Let children know that the song is about a letter written to a loved one who died.

- Invite children to make up a song about their loved one who died or to sing the favorite song of a person they knew who died.

- Read *The Wall* by Eve Bunting. Explain that some people who are famous or who have been helpful to many others have monuments honoring them after death.

Feeling Sorrow

Introduce and explain the word *sympathy* to children. Read a few sympathy cards to them and talk about what they mean. Select cards that express emotion without representing specific religions. Let children know that some people send sympathy cards to friends when someone they love dies but not everyone follows this practice. Assure children that most people feel really sad when someone they love dies, and the sympathy cards let them know that a friend is thinking about them.

MATERIALS
- a variety of sympathy cards

OTHER IDEAS

- Read *I Miss You: A First Look at Death* by Pat Thomas. Help children identify *missing* as one of the many emotions we feel when someone we love dies.

- Read *Nana Upstairs & Nana Downstairs* by Tomie dePaola. Let children know that telling stories about someone you love who dies can help you feel better.

- Read and discuss *My Hands Sing the Blues: Romare Bearden's Childhood Journey* by Jeanne Walker Harvey.

- Talk with children about how some people express their emotions by telling stories or painting, and others express their emotions by singing. To follow up, play selected blues music.

- Share with children that some people believe they should celebrate the time they had with a loved one who dies. One way to celebrate is to laugh. Encourage children to offer special "giggle stories" to the group about any pet, friend, or relative who has died.

The Cemetery

Arrange for children to take a field trip to a cemetery (human or pet) where a burial is about to take place or has recently taken place. In advance, prepare children about proper cemetery etiquette, and remind them frequently during the visit to be respectful. If possible, watch a grave being dug, and talk about how deep they think it is. Assist children in measuring the size of the plots and the size of headstones or other markers. Encourage children to examine headstones and look for familiar letters in the epitaph before you read it to them. Point out the dates, and let children know how old the person was when he or she died and how many years ago the death occurred. Suggest that children look at the flowers, artwork on headstones, benches, statues, and monuments. Look to see what other buildings are on the grounds, such as an office, chapel, grounds maintenance facility, or mausoleum. Let children know that some families do not use cemeteries.

MATERIALS

- a measuring tape

OTHER IDEAS

- Arrange for a field trip to a funeral home, or watch a video clip that shows children rooms where funerals are held, guest books, sample programs, obituaries, coffins, a hearse, and other physical objects associated with funerals. Listen to examples of music played at funerals. Explain to children that some people believe in having funerals or memorial services and others do not. Be sure to help them understand that even those who have funerals may have very different kinds.

- Ask a florist to demonstrate how to arrange flowers, and show sample photographs of arrangements for funerals, memorial services, or gravesites. Ask the florist for a donation of old flowers, or provide artificial flowers for children to make arrangements. Consider delivering the arrangement to a local family, with sympathy from the class.

- Provide materials for children to making rubbings of gravestones using aluminum foil or paper and charcoal. Remind children to be respectful by leaving the gravestone as they found it and the site free of their supplies.

Life and Death

Show children seed packets for flowers and vegetables. Divide the children into small groups, and let each group select seeds to plant. Support each group in gathering information about when and how to grow their selection. Each group will begin with two pots of planted seeds. One pot will be given light, water, and attention. The other plant will be deprived of sufficient light and water once it has sprouted. Encourage children to frequently measure and record the plant growth (or lack of it) and to take photographs or make drawings of their plants at various stages. Children will see their plant dying and will examine it during the process.

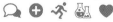

MATERIALS

- flower and vegetable seeds, pots, a watering container, soil, a measuring device (ruler, yardstick), a camera, and lighting for indoor plants (a grow light or a fluorescent light)

OTHER IDEAS

- Visit a nearby farm, field, park, or your program grounds during various times of the year, and take photographs and document on a chart what things are living, growing, being planted, harvested, dormant, or dead.
  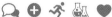

- Visit a garden center or plant nursery, and learn about the job of caring for plants. Ask to see plants in all stages of life and death.

- Read and discuss *Watching the Seasons* by Edana Eckart.

- Provide nonpoisonous houseplants in ailing conditions, and support children in trying to nurse the plants back to health. Celebrate when plants become healthy, and help children understand and accept their lack of success at improving the health of some plants.
  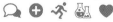

FAMILY INFORMATION

WHEN SOMEONE OR SOMETHING SPECIAL TO ME DIES

Death of a loved one, a classmate, or a much loved pet can be traumatic. When a person or pet dies, your child may experience various emotions, depending on her or his age and development and on how close he or she was to the person or animal.

A child may be sad, angry, scared, or confused. Sometimes children seem unconcerned or even happy. Children do not always have the same feelings as adults, and they may show their emotions in different ways. Talk with your child about feelings and how feelings can be shown.

TALK WITH YOUR CHILD

Children often have difficulty understanding that the deceased person or pet will not return. They see characters in cartoons, television programs, and movies portrayed as dead or dying, yet those characters appear the next day or week in a new program. Young children may not comprehend that situations they view through media may not be real.

The rituals associated with death may be comforting, or they may confuse or frighten a child. Encourage your child to ask questions. Answer those questions honestly and to the best of your ability. If you do not know the answer, it is okay to say, "I don't know. What do you think?" Explore your family beliefs and knowledge with your child.

It may help children to gather pictures of deceased relatives and discuss what you remember about them. If you attended funerals or ceremonies for the relatives, describe what took place.

FAMILY ACTIVITY

Cut out the following pictures, and assist your child in placing each set in the order of the life cycle of the tree and flowers represented. Begin a discussion about how plants, people, pets, and all living things are born, grow, and die. If a family pet, a close relative, or a friend has died recently, encourage your child to talk about her or his feelings, sense of loss, and grief. You may wish to begin discussing ways to honor and remember special people and pets who have died.

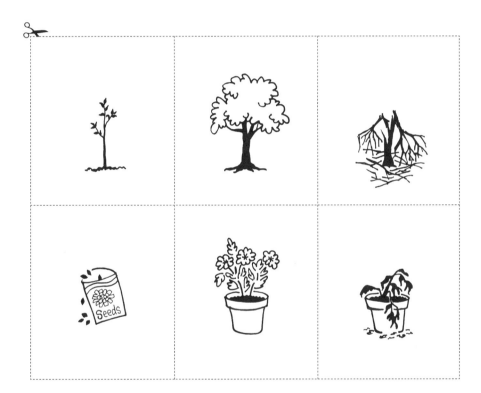